Fall asleep!

It's Easy...

The (miraculous)

Kaleidoscope Method

How to get to sleep, sleep help, sleep problems, how to cure Insomnia and have better sleep

By Elli Yeates

Please review this book

so you can help other people to sleep!

I would love your feedback

If you have questions or comments or you want to know more, then you can contact me:

http://helpmetosleepblog.wordpress.com

Table of Contents

CHAPTER 01

INTRODUCTION

What will this book do for you? This book will put you to sleep...... It is going to teach you **exactly how** to go to sleep in 5 simple steps using a brand new technique: The Kaleidoscope Method. It's *that* simple; read it today and sleep tonight. You will find it quick and easy to read and understand, so you *really* will be able to read it *now* and use the steps you have just learnt *tonight* to go to sleep.

The Kaleidoscope method is completely natural and free of drugs. It is easy and accessible to anyone. In fact it is almost as if this technique has rested in our heads for ever but we just hadn't put two and two together to realize its potential.

Who is it for? Anyone who either: has trouble getting off to sleep *or* wakes in the night and cannot get back to sleep, is going to learn **exactly how** to fall, or fall back to sleep. You will have a simple process to follow **that works**!

What won't this book do? It won't stop you snoring or prevent sleep apnoea and it won't cure any underlying medical conditions that make sleeping difficult. It may not stop you from waking through the night. However, it *will* teach you a way to get *back* to sleep even if you are being woken numerous times through the night. Once you are taught exactly *how* to get back to sleep, waking up during the night isn't nearly as annoying or traumatic.

Does this sound familiar?

I'm awake......Oh no, that's not good...what time is it? It's 2:15am....didn't I wake up at this exact time last night? I have a huge day tomorrow......I bet I won't be able to get back to sleep....Just like last night, I finally fell asleep 30minutes before the alarm went off..... Now I'm going to be exhausted and have red eyes and black rings under them......I need to sleep!!!!...Hmmm, have I done everything for tomorrow .....I'm sure I was meant to contact someone else......No, stop thinking, go to sleep!!......I could get up and take a tablet – but I did that twice last week...this is starting to be a habit, besides they make me feel horrible....Sleeping is meant to be easy; What is wrong with me????

Rest assured, there is *nothing* wrong with you. Sleeping problems are unbelievably common. For some reason we seem to have lost our ability to drift off to sleep and stay there until we are well rested in the morning.

Now that our lives are *so* demanding, requiring huge levels of organisation and countless decisions to be made every hour we need more than ever to be firing on all cylinders *every* waking hour. We need our sleep!

Whether you lie in bed for hours not being able to drift off, or wake in the middle of the night and toss and turn until morning, the net effect is the same: exhaustion, poor decision making, a feeling of despair and ill health.

The Kaleidoscope method:

You are about to reset your body and learn *exactly how* to fall asleep – at the start of the night, in the middle of the night or 1 hour before dawn.

It's easy and quick – you will be able to do it tonight and from now on, until sleeping really is EASY and ENJOYABLE!

Before I start, let me tell you a little bit about how all this began……….

I am 47 years old, I work full time as a school teacher and I am a great sleeper!!

It wasn't always this way. I didn't start having problems

with sleep until I was about 25. It crept up gradually and got worse and worse. Although I was really tired I just couldn't drop off to sleep. What had once been a hugely enjoyable part of the day; when I got to slide into bed, forget all my troubles and drift off became a battle ground.

I had always been such a good sleeper! How could this be happening? I started to get quite worried and tense about going to sleep and would dread the whole process. This of course just made matters worse.

One night, quite by accident I discovered what I have named the **Kaleidoscope Method**. It worked and I went off to sleep and didn't wake until morning. At first I didn't realize what I had discovered because, when you think about it, you don't actually remember the moment you fall asleep. Eventually it hit me; those rather fun steps that I thought of as a game were actually sending me to sleep! Since then I have used the

Kaleidoscope method every time I have had trouble sleeping; at the start of the night, in the middle of the night or one hour before dawn and it has worked every single time!

I'm not sure what sets you off, but for me whenever I wake in the middle of the night my mind takes over and I start worrying and thinking about stupid things. As soon as I realize what I am doing I start the simple Kaleidoscope process and before I know it, it is morning and I have obviously gone straight back to sleep.

For quite a while I would let myself indulge in a few hours of worrying and obsessing about my problems or thoughts. After all, it is nice and quiet and there is no one to disturb you from your thinking. But eventually I decided that about 90% of the thoughts I had in the middle of the night were ridiculous and a complete waste of valuable sleep time!

Have you ever noticed that the problems you spend hours worrying about in the dead of night seem silly or easily solved when you think about them in the morning? What's more, after a good night's sleep you are far more able to think clearly and logically.

So, what I do now is sleep really well at night and do all my problem solving during the day. And I tell you what; it is a way more effective way of living your life! When I wake up in the middle of the night I have to take control and say to myself; 'These stupid thoughts are a waste of time, I am ready for sleep, time for the Kaleidoscope method'. And that's usually the last thing I remember before waking in the morning.

It really is that easy! The only difficult thing is making the *decision* that what you really need is sleep, not thinking time, and then following through with the Kaleidoscope method.

The other thing I have noticed is that getting to sleep using this method gets faster and faster each time you do it! That's right, it's a short process anyhow, but the more you do it, the better you get. Imagine being able to wake in the middle of the night, look at the clock and not groan! Instead you can think, 'Wow, three more hours sleep, how lucky am I?!'

If you have been checked out by a medical practitioner and there are no medical reasons for your sleep problems then this book is going to give you a simple process to follow that will send you off to sleep – in the middle of the night, at the beginning of the night or 1 hour before you have to get up! What's more it will give you a confident attitude to sleeping because you will know that even if you do wake up you can get back to sleep quickly no matter what time it is. All that anxiety is taken away.

So, get ready for your sleeping problems to dissolve!

Just a word of warning: don't be tempted to jump straight to the Kaleidoscope chapter without reading the pages before it. Although you may have read some of this information before it is important that you eliminate any possible factor that may be aggravating your sleeping problems.

CHAPTER 02

WHAT ARE THE
BENEFITS OF SLEEP?

If you have had trouble getting a good night's sleep then you will know that sleep really affects your ability to function the next day, but did you know that.....

- A lack of sleep causes inflammation and puts your body into a state of stress. Your blood pressure increases and you are more likely to suffer from heart attack, stroke, diabetes and cancer.

- Sleep keeps you healthy because it reduces blood pressure and is a time when your body builds and repairs cells. A lack of sleep increases blood pressure which accelerates the degeneration of body cells and causes premature ageing

- Sleep improves your memory. While you are asleep your brain consolidates and links memories and makes connections. If you are trying to operate normally after a poor night's sleep you will be less alert and will have an uphill battle remembering people's names, conversations or even basic facts.

- A lack of sleep will prevent you from processing and understanding new information the next day. What's more it is vital to get a good night's sleep after you have learnt new information to ensure it is remembered.

- A lack of sleep is associated with obesity and over-weight. The body hormones that regulate appetite are unbalanced by a lack of sleep and this is why people who get less than 7 hours of sleep a night are more likely to be overweight or obese.

- A lack of sleep can make you moody the next day, but in the long term a chronic lack of sleep can lead to depression and anxiety.

So, not only is difficulty sleeping *extremely* annoying and exhausting for the sufferer there are many well documented studies telling us that it is also a *serious problem* that is detrimental to our health.

CHAPTER 03

WHAT WILL HELP AND WHAT SHOULD I AVOID?

Make sure you **read this list well**. Don't be tempted to skip this part because quite often you might be unknowingly doing something that will make sleep more difficult for you.

- Avoid afternoon sleeps. It is so tempting, if you are able, to have a snooze in the quiet of the afternoon, especially if you have slept badly the night before. This is not a good idea! Whilst it feels fabulous at the time you are going to pay for it in the middle of the night when you are wide awake. The only exception to this rule is if you are able to confidently take a 20 minute power nap without it extending any longer than that.

- Have a regular bedtime and wake time each day. Keeping your body in a regular rhythm will mean you are going to be tired at the right times.

- Watch your consumption of caffeine in coffee, cola drinks and high caffeine drinks. Any time you consume more than normal you are more likely to have trouble sleeping. Many people adjust to consuming a certain amount of caffeine each day but if they increase that amount will immediately notice an impact on their sleeping habits.

- Limit your consumption of alcohol! 'But it makes me sleepy' you say? That's true, it may send you off to sleep effectively but... you will more often than not wake sometime during the night and be wide awake unable to return to that blissful state. Best policy is to stop drinking alcohol a couple of hours before your normal bed time. Have plenty of water and make sure you are feeling sober before sleep.

- Make sure that you have checked your medications with your Medical Practitioner to rule out those as a cause of your insomnia. This is especially important if you have suddenly developed sleeping problems; it may coincide with a new or change in medication.

CHAPTER 04

WHEN SHOULD I USE IT?

There is nothing wrong with using the Kaleidoscope method every time you want to go to sleep. This could include:

- At your normal sleep time

- When you have woken in the middle of the night

- When you have woken a bit too early and you want an extra hour's sleep before the alarm is going to go off in the morning

- On a plane or train when you are travelling through a sleep time

When you use the Kaleidoscope method will vary for each person. If you *only* have problems with waking in the middle of the night and not being able to get back to sleep, then save the Kaleidoscope method for only those times. Use your usual method for going to sleep at the beginning of the night.

If you find that after 20 minutes that your usual method of falling asleep isn't working then it is time to start the Kaleidoscope steps.

Some nights there may be something on your mind and this will be keeping you awake. This is definitely a time for the Kaleidoscope method. You are far better off thinking things through in daylight hours after a long restful sleep than tossing and turning and reaching wild conclusions in the middle of the night.

If you regularly wake up during the night to go to the bathroom, let the cat out, attend to a baby etc. then these are great times to use the Kaleidoscope steps. If possible keep the lights off or really dim when you get up, try to only open your eyes as much as is necessary and don't start thinking! When you get back to bed immediately begin the Kaleidoscope steps. With a bit of practise you will find that you can now easily get back to sleep even if you are woken several times during the night.

I like to challenge myself – for instance, when I wake up 45 minutes before the alarm to see if I can get back to sleep. And guess what? I have an almost 100% success rate – unless I am not really committed because I am eager to start the day.

CHAPTER 05

STEP ONE – GET READY

Now that you have read all the previous chapters this one is about how to set yourself up for success. It is the start of the 5 steps, and each one is of equal importance and should be done in order.

It may seem a bit much, but I suggest that you start planning for your night' sleep at the **beginning** of the day:

- Make sure you have done some exercise if at all possible during the day, preferably early in the day. This is going to help your body feel physically tired and in need of sleep. (By the way, avoid exercise within a few hours of your sleep time as it might have the opposite effect and keep you awake)

- Do not lie around in bed during the day and do not have a little afternoon nap

- Try and have your evening meal at least 3 hours before you go to sleep to avoid problems with indigestion and an uncomfortably full stomach

- Plan your bed time and try to stick to it and not get side tracked by your computer, phone or TV. There is no point going to bed an hour earlier than normal because you are probably not going to feel tired. Stick to a regular routine and aim for a quality night's sleep that does not include hours of waking

- Make sure you have stopped drinking alcohol well before your allocated bed time so that you are feeling sober

- An hour before your bedtime start dimming the lights to send signals to your body that it is time to start slowing down

- Try *really* hard not to let yourself fall asleep in front of the TV. What usually happens is that you fall into a delicious, deep sleep on the couch, but once you wake up and get to the bedroom you will either be wide awake or you will fall asleep for a short while but then be wide wake in the middle of the night

- If you like to have a hot drink before bed try to have drunk this an hour before your bed time so that you don't have to get up to the bathroom a couple of hours in to your sleep

- Check the temperature of your room, clothing and bed coverings. Being too cold or too hot will wake you up and make it difficult to get back to sleep. If you have ever looked after a baby you will know how true this is

- Make your bed a nice place to be: wash the coverings; make it carefully so that nothing is going to irritate you during the night

- Put your phone, laptop or device in another room so that you cannot hear it making little noises that indicate you should look at it

- If you often wake in the night and remember something crucially important then put a pen and paper near the bed so you can scribble it down when it occurs to you. This will allow you to let it go and be able to go back to sleep

- Check for dripping taps, ticking clocks, annoying lights and excess noise. Try and deal with these as best as possible *before* sleep

- Have a clock with illuminated numbers near you, but not shining on you, so that if you wake you can quickly satisfy your curiosity as to what time it is.

- Have a water bottle near your bed so you can take a quick sip if you wake up thirsty without having to sit up or turn on a light.

- Have a box of tissues near your bed if you know you will need to blow your nose.

- Go to the bathroom just before getting in to bed

Ok, you are ready for bed and step 2!

Chapter 06

Step Two – Get Comfy

Ok, you are in your super comfortable bed and everything is just right! Now what?

It's time to position yourself correctly in bed and get your breathing right.

Your sleeping position is important. Don't worry too

much about what you have read is the best sleeping position. Instead, think about what position you are in when you *usually* fall off to sleep and choose that one. Chances are that you will have the most success with your *old favourite* position.

Get your pillow, if you are using one, just right. Fix up the bed coverings and get your arms and legs in a relaxing position that can be maintained for the whole night. I like to sleep flat on my back with my arms by my sides and legs straight. You are going to need to be as still as possible so make sure it is a position you can maintain.

Now start breathing through your nose. Don't worry too much about your breathing; you won't have to concentrate on it other than setting up regular breaths in and out through your nose.

Ok, that was easy, now you are ready for step 3...

CHAPTER 07

STEP THREE: THE DECISION

You don't always have to use the Kaleidoscope method to get off to sleep. If you have another method that works well (and you are reading this because you wake during the night) then use your usual method and save the Kaleidoscope method until the middle of the night when you can't drop back off.

If you like to read, or listen to music, that is fine too. Generally 10-30 minutes of reading or music should be enough before sleep.

Once you have truly started your usual sleep process and it is not working after about 20 minutes then it is time to move on to step three.

You may have discovered something that is annoying you for example you think you may need to visit the bathroom, or the cat is meowing to be let in, or there is a light shining in your eye. Whatever the problem, get up, trying to keep your eyes fairly closed, turn on as few lights as possible and attend to the problem.

Return to bed and assume your comfortable position covered in step 2.

Ok, now you are ready for step 3. At this point you will have spent some time trying to go to sleep or you have woken in the middle of the night. You may have found that instead of sleep you are doing a re-run of the day's events, or a planning session of tomorrow's events, or you may be working through a random list of things to worry about.

If you have woken in the middle of the night with a sudden, important thought write it down with that pen and paper you prepared earlier so that you can put it out of your mind and get back to sleep.

At this point you need to come to the realization that whatever your mind is thinking about it is unlikely to be very sensible or productive at this hour. You need to actively say to yourself, 'that is enough, I need to get to sleep/back to sleep and any thoughts I am having now will be much better thought through tomorrow after a great night's sleep.'

In fact, this is *the most important step* of all because you are actively **committing** yourself to the Kaleidoscope steps. Whenever I have trouble getting to sleep or back to sleep it is almost *always* because I have not really made a commitment to the process. I will have become so involved in whatever I am thinking about that I am not actually *trying* to go to sleep. However, once I acknowledge this is what I am doing, and make the *decision* to sleep, then the Kaleidoscope method always works.

So that is it, step 3 is all about *admitting* that you are not falling asleep and actively making the decision that you will commit yourself to the Kaleidoscope steps…. no more mucking around. It is time for sleep and time for **step 4, The Onscreen Kaleidoscope.**

Chapter 08

Step Four:

The Onscreen Kaleidoscope

You should be in your comfortable sleeping position with arms and legs relaxed. Make sure you are breathing through your nose and keep your body really still. Avoid the temptation to stretch or change positions.

Close your eyes and when they are shut concentrate on the lights that you can see when your eyes are shut. Let me explain...

What are these lights? They are called Phosphenes. More specifically they are entopic. This means it is light you see when there is no light actually entering the eye. When you gently rub or move your closed eyes you are stimulating the cells in the Retina making your brain think that you are seeing light and making it behave in a similar way.

Some people will know exactly what I am talking about and may have spent many a childhood hour rubbing their closed eyes and delighting in the patterns that result. Others will be less sure and will need to do a bit of a practice.

If you are having trouble seeing these lights, don't worry because the more you look the more you will see. Before

trying this in bed, try it in a
well-lit room when you are not
about to go to sleep so you
know you will be able to do it
later. Try it now. Close your
eyes and then rub them gently
if necessary. You should see a
moving array of bright lights
that fade and change and
appear and disappear. Try it
again, but instead of rubbing
your eyes simply move your
eyeballs slowly behind your
closed eyelids or blink without
opening your eyes. You won't
get such a dramatic effect as
when rubbing but moving your
eyeballs or closed–eye blinking

are the **preferred methods** because you don't have to move your arms and hands to get the effect. You want to be able to keep your whole body as still as possible during this step and the next because that will help you get to sleep.

Once you have practised using the Kaleidoscope method you won't have trouble seeing the lights, they will jump out at you as soon as you close your eyes! In the meantime close your eyes and then slowly move your eyeballs around. If that really doesn't work at all then gently squeeze your shut eyes.

Once you have found the lights in front of your shut eyes you will notice that they are a bit like a Kaleidoscope, in that they keep moving around and changing. Just like a Kaleidoscope they are quite entertaining to watch. Let yourself become totally absorbed in their movement, watch them change, brighten, disappear and reappear. Some people see colour, others black and white. I pretty much always see black and white. I am always amazed at how different they can be no matter how many times I have done it. It is also like watching a computer screen. You can actually decide to zoom in to see more detail and to watch the lights changing from one shape to another. This is why have termed it the onscreen Kaleidoscope. It looks like a Kaleidoscope and you can zoom in just like a computer screen filling up your entire vision.

After finding the lights and following them for a little while your brain will start thinking about something else, re-enacting a conversation from the day or thinking about an upcoming event or in fact a million different possible distractions!

As soon as you realize that is what you are doing, recognise it; "woops I've drifted off" and find the lights again and become reabsorbed. Don't be surprised if you have to do this over and over again. You will watch the lights for a little while, become distracted by some other thought, realize what you are doing and then actively go back to looking at the Kaleidoscope. Don't get frustrated with yourself or angry at the amount of times you get distracted because so long as you keep going back to the Onscreen Kaleidoscope the whole process is putting you to sleep. Keep your mood happy and positive but just keep concentrating on the Kaleidoscope for as long as you can and immediately stop yourself when you notice you have been distracted.

Sometimes you will be able to tell you are starting to fall asleep but usually it just happens and you won't remember a thing. One sure sign that the process is working is that you will realize that you can no longer sense your feet and most of your legs. If this happens just smile to yourself and quickly get back to admiring that Kaleidoscope. Whatever you do, try to avoid stretching to get feeling back in those legs or changing sleep positions. This will just be unsettling and mean you have to go through that whole process again.

The main focus for step four is to find and follow the Onscreen Kaleidoscope. Focus and become enchanted with the wonderful patterns that are being created in front of you. It's almost as if the technique for going to sleep has been provided for us but no one has realized it is right there! Be ready for distraction and

lol.
yes.

instead of getting frustrated when it happens just acknowledge that it has happened and go straight back to the lights. Remember *it doesn't matter* how many times you are distracted so long as you are actively trying to stay concentrating on the Kaleidoscope and immediately go back to it once you realize you are thinking about something else. It is this *process* that will put you to sleep.

The Kaleidoscope IS a distraction.

You will not fall asleep by cheating the system and trying to maintain a vague picture of lights in your head while you are really thinking about something else.

All you should be thinking is something like this little dialogue: "where are the lights?... ah there they are.. there aren't many.. ah now there are more... oh look, that is amazing... that looks like feathers, oh now it is a huge flower....where does this series of lights go?...it feels like a roller coaster"…….. and so on.

This type of dialogue with yourself will be about the last thing you remember before you fall asleep……

Chapter 09

Step Five – Get back to it

If something happens during Step Four and you get completely woken or distracted then you may have to quickly go back a few steps in readiness for sleep.

Don't get into a panic or get angry, just make sure you are comfortable.

If you are hot or cold make sure you change bedclothes or room temperature to fix this.

If you now realize you need to go to the bathroom or put the cat out, try to do it by turning on as few lights as possible. Even try to keep your eyes mostly closed, without crashing into things of course!

Have a sip of water if your mouth is dry or jot down that thought if it is really worrying you.

You should get back to Step 3 and make sure your sleeping position is comfortable and that you are breathing through your nose. Remember use the position that you usually fall asleep in. The temptation to change positions is strong but you will tend to fall asleep in your favourite position. The only time I allow myself to change positions is when I can feel I am really close to falling asleep and I have an overwhelming desire to turn.

Stay calm. You have a process to follow and it will work.

Find the Onscreen Kaleidoscope and allow yourself to be intrigued and entertained by it.

Acknowledge your distractions and quickly get back to the Kaleidoscope.

You will find that with a bit of practise once you feel yourself waking up during the night, instead of checking the time you will immediately look for the Kaleidoscope and start falling back to sleep *before* you have had a chance to really wake up.

You will soon realize that even if you wake up 40 minutes before your alarm you *will* be able to go back to sleep using the Kaleidoscope method.

Keep in mind that if you stay calm, enjoy the Onscreen Kaleidoscope and accept that you will be distracted, the whole process is faster and you will fall asleep more quickly than if you get discouraged or frustrated each time your thoughts wonder off.

If you are having a really bad night it is usually because you have not committed yourself to Step 3: The Decision. Once you are worked up thinking about a problem, issue, or event that dominates your thinking you really need to take control and make *the decision* that it is time to sleep and to start the Kaleidoscope method. If ever I struggle to fall asleep it is always because I am excited or worried about something and in truth I have not committed myself to the sleeping process. Once I commit myself to **the decision** and start the steps, it always works.

If you have been living through a long built up pattern of poor sleeping habits then you may find that it takes you longer to fall asleep the first time you use the Kaleidoscope steps than it will take you after a bit of practice. Your body clock may have almost set its self into a pattern of being awake for several hours at the start or in the middle of the night. But don't worry; it will be quite happy to readjust to a more normal sleep pattern once you have a strategy to follow.

So, be patient, follow the Kaleidoscope steps; it **will** work. Your body might put up a bit of a fight at first but you will find that the process gets faster and faster until waking during the night or falling asleep is no longer an issue.......
and sleep is now deeply pleasurable and restorative as it should be

CHAPTER 10

WOW, THAT MUST HAVE WORKED!

The funny thing about the Kaleidoscope method for me was that it took a while to realize that watching those lights was actually sending me to sleep. Why? Because I fell deliciously asleep and didn't think about it in the morning!

It took a little while before I made the association between the Onscreen Kaleidoscope and falling asleep! Once I realized what I had discovered I starting trying to test the method. Would it work at the start of the night, in the middle of the night, half an hour before I had to get up?

So long as I followed all the other steps religiously then it worked every time. And it will for you too!

Remember, plan your sleeping early – check that you have

followed all the guidelines presented in *Chapter 3: Things to avoid and things that will help.* You cannot expect to have a normal night's sleep if you have had two extra caffeine drinks during the day or you have had a 90-minute afternoon sleep.

Once you have set your day up for a good night's sleep then it is time to follow the Kaleidoscope steps:

Step One: Get ready – your room and bed are conducive to sleeping, it's your normal bed time, you didn't fall asleep in front of the TV, electronic equipment is away, you are sober and ready for sleep

Step Two: Get comfy – you are in your favourite sleeping position; breathing in and out through your nose

Step Three: The decision – you have made a conscious *decision* that it is time to sleep and that you are committed to the Kaleidoscope steps

Step Four: The Onscreen Kaleidoscope – you have found the lights and you are absorbed by watching them

Step Five: Get back to it – as soon as you become distracted (and you will) you quickly and calmly get back to the Onscreen Kaleidoscope and keep repeating steps 4 and 5 until you are asleep

You may find that in the middle of the night you may need to go to the bathroom and have to go right back to step one and start the steps from the beginning. Remember try not to turn on lights or open your eyes too much. Once you are back in bed you can quickly start the process again and get back to sleep.

Remember the more you do this process the faster it becomes!

Sleep is no longer going to be a trauma; instead a pleasure! You have steps to follow and they *will* work. It is such a relief to have a process to follow when you wake up in the middle of the night or when you can't get to sleep. A simple process takes away all the anxiety and stress and allows you to concentrate on the steps alone, instead of the 500 other things that you are thinking about.

CHAPTER 11

WHERE TO FROM HERE?

Once you learn the Kaleidoscope method you will be set for a life of luxurious sleeping.

If it doesn't work on any occasion try to work out which step you haven't followed. Maybe you had an extra coffee during the day and this has kept you awake, maybe you indulged in a bit of midnight worrying and didn't really give the Kaleidoscope Steps your best effort?

You will find the method gets really easy to follow with a bit of practise. The steps start to merge into one process that you will learn to follow diligently. Eventually you will probably come to the same realization as me, and that is that *The Decision* is the most important step of all. That is when you actively take control of your brain and insist that sleep must follow.

Remember that the Kaleidoscope Method is not going to cure any other underlying medical problems that may be interrupting your sleep. However, it *will* give you a process to follow each time you wake that will *teach* you how to get back to sleep.

The very knowledge that you are able to get to sleep when the time is right is so relieving that a lot of your sleep problems may disappear as a consequence. Instead of waking in the middle of the night and immediately being overcome with anxiety at the thought of not being able to get back to sleep, you will instead simply stretch and yawn, look for the Kaleidoscope and go straight back to sleep. Learning these steps is truly liberating. Your sleep time will be yours again to enjoy.

So, what should you do now?

First of all try finding the Kaleidoscope during the day, when you are not trying to fall off to sleep. If you can see it now you will have no trouble during the night.

Next, make sure you have set your day up for a good night's sleep by checking the *Things to avoid and things that will help* list in Chapter 3.

Go through the Kaleidoscope Steps 1-5 and make sure you

remember the process, without leaving anything out.

The steps are really quite simple and Chapter 10 has a very brief summary to refresh your memory. The idea is to read the book, learn the process and then try it out when you are going to sleep at night. You are not meant to have the book next to your bed and be turning the light on and off checking each step!

This would most definitely make sleeping more difficult!

When you wake up each morning make yourself think back to the night before. Did you get to sleep easily? Did you wake up during the night? How many times? Do you remember using the Kaleidoscope steps? It is very reassuring when you realize that you did use the steps and that they *must* have worked because you don't remember anything else!

Get the most out of your life! Enjoy your sleeping.........every night for the rest of your life.

Made in the USA
Lexington, KY
29 December 2012